THE SECRET LIFE OF YOUR BLOOD SUGAR

A DIABETES SKELETON
IN YOUR DOCTOR'S CLOSET

Kfir Luzzatto, Ph.D.

PINE 10

Pine Ten, LLC
500 N Michigan Ave.
Chicago, IL 60611

The author of this book does not dispense medical advice or prescribe the use of any technique as a form of treatment for physical, emotional or medical problems without the advice of a physician, either directly or indirectly. The intent of the author is only to offer information of a general nature. In the event that you use any of the information in this book for yourself, which is your constitutional right, the author and the publisher assume no responsibility for your actions.

Fist publication, August 2017

ISBN-10: 1-938212-46-0
ISBN-13: 978-1-938212-46-8

Contents

Introduction

Some people are good at looking the other way when their body tells them that something is wrong with them. I had being doing it successfully for quite some time, but come March of 2016, I could no longer ignore the fact that I wasn't feeling well. My doctor recommended an extensive blood test, which came back on March 10 and ruined my day (and much of my life after that). My fasting plasma glucose level (FPG) (affectionately called "blood sugar") was 312 mg/dl—way above the recommended level of 100—and my HbA1C (which tells you how your blood sugar level has been doing in the past three months or so) was at an astronomic 12.1% (the maximum recommended level of a healthy person being 5.7%).

With those numbers, I had to do something immediately, or I was in line for hideous diseases and premature death. My doctor immediately placed me on strong medication. As a result, only three months later, on June 21, 2016, my fasting blood sugar level had dropped to 138 mg/dl and my HbA1C to a mere 6%. That's great, right? **Wrong**!

Fast forward eight months to February 14, 2017. My fasting blood sugar level had gone up to 157 mg/dl, and my HbA1C to 6.8%. The efficacy of the treatment was obviously diminishing, and I started to recall people telling me that, once you start on the path of blood sugar medication, you may end up injecting insulin. I wasn't going to take that lying down.

When you become diabetic, you want to think that it is an Act of God, that you are not responsible for it. It's just the world being mean to you. But while obviously in some cases diabetes may be due to your genetic makeup or to other causes over which you have no control, that's untrue for most people. The reading and reasoning that I had done over the months since that fateful morning in March had convinced me that I had been causing it to myself with my own hands. I had been overeating and, what's worse, eating the wrong kinds of food. I was overweight and wasn't exercising enough. I reasoned that what I did to myself I might perhaps undo, if I could just find and follow the right path.

It took me five more months to prove that I was right and that managing my blood sugar level without taking drugs was possible. After stopping taking medication altogether for three and a half months (after a thorough, responsible, and careful priming period), I took a new blood test, on July 19, 2017. My fasting blood sugar was 102 mg/dl and my HbA1C was 5.8%. I'll say it again: **I'm taking no medication!** If you read on, I'll share my test results with you in detail.

I'm not going to tell you that what I did was easy and required no effort. But if you haven't ruined your pancreas for good and you follow my example with perseverance and motivation, you may be able to accomplish the same result that I did, or even better. Hundreds of people that I know of have done the same. This appears to be the best-kept secret of the medical profession: In the majority of cases you can rid yourself of type 2 diabetes.

That doesn't mean that at that point you will be able to start wolfing down sugar again like there's no tomorrow, mind you. It means that you can lead a satisfactory life, remaining mindful of what you eat and how you run your day, without feeling that you are missing out on anything.

In tackling my problem I had the help of a coach, to whom I'll give due credit in the pages to follow, but most people don't have access to someone like him. When you embark on a completely new endeavor, venturing into uncharted territories, it is extremely helpful to have someone who resolves your doubts and tells you which way to go—even if at times he is wrong. Going in the wrong direction and learning that what you did is not for you, is way better than remaining frozen, undecided on what to do. A conclusion that eating this or that is not what you need is important data, and managing your problem is all about having the right data. Once you have sufficient data, you are on the right path.

As I will discuss further in the next few chapters, where managing your blood sugar level is concerned, there is no universal truth. No magic formula exists that works for everybody, because everybody is different. That's why you must be your own body explorer and find your own very personal solution. The only help that a coach can give you is to point you in the right direction, giving you some information that is universally applicable, and prompting you to discover the remaining, non-universal rules that apply specifically to you. The aim of this book is to fill that role, to provide information, useful tips, and, especially, the encouragement that everybody needs while pursuing the solitary task of getting better.

If you have the will, the determination and the stamina needed to beat type 2 diabetes, turn the page. And if you don't have them, go pop another pill and may God be with you, because if you don't help yourself, only He can help you.

CHAPTER 1
How to Start

You have been diagnosed with type 2 diabetes and have decided to fight back, otherwise you wouldn't be reading this book. But how does one embark on the path that, hopefully, will end the dependency on glucose-lowering drugs? I can't tell you what exactly will work best for you, because we are all different, but what I can do is to tell you, in all the details, how *I* did it. I believe that everyone should find his or her own exact path to success, but knowing the direction in which to go and what has worked for others, is a basis on which you can build. I know it, because that's what I did, as I will relate in a minute.

I am a chemical engineer, a patent attorney, an inventor, and a thriller writer (not necessarily in that order) and, as such, I enjoy a broad vision of many fields. This is particularly true because I have been working closely on medical subjects for many more years than I care to remember, and have absorbed a vast body of information. As I already mentioned in another book[1], sometimes the distance between success and failure is simply knowing that success is possible. Belief is a powerful driving force that empowers you to do deeds you never

---

[1] Do It With Words: Regrow Your Hair with Your Mind

thought you would dare to attempt. Knowing (or believing) that it is possible to achieve an ambitious goal empowers gifted scientists to accomplish results previously thought to be out of reach. It was the same for me: I rid myself of the need for medication (my current results, give or take a line or two, are those of a healthy individual) simply because I believed it was possible and took steps to act on that belief. By telling you all about it, in minute detail, I am making it possible for you too, and now it is up to you to decide whether you want to follow my example and become your own body explorer.

As a motivational aid, please take a look at what happened to my fasting glucose levels (Fig. 1) and HbA1C levels (Fig. 2), keeping in mind that I stopped taking glucose-lowering medication on April 4, 2017 (dates in the tables are in the DD/MM/YY format):

Fig. 1: Fasting Glucose Levels.
Source: Kfir's Maccabi[2] Healthcare Online Records

102 mg/dl	19-07-2017
157 mg/dl	14-02-2017
138 mg/dl	07-08-2016
312 mg/dl	10-03-2016

---

[2] Maccabi Healthcare Services is a leading Israeli Health Fund

Fig. 2: HbA1C Levels.
Source: Kfir's Maccabi Healthcare Online Records

5.8 % Total Hb.	19-07-2017
6.8 % Total Hb.	14-02-2017
6 % Total Hb.	21-06-2016
12.1 % Total Hb.	10-03-2016

Our body is a highly sophisticated, incredibly complex chemical plant. An unbelievable number of chemical reactions are taking place in our body at every moment, even as you read these words and need to flip the page, move your eyes, or simply store the information you are receiving. As a chemical engineer, I am well aware that if you try to make a given product without feeding the correct raw material to the plant, you are not going to get it. That started a train of thought about the level of control that we have on what our body does, by feeding it the right "raw materials," as well as the role of our mind in telling the "chemical plant" in our body what to do with the raw material that is available to it (which I will discuss in Chapter 5). Given my conclusion that it is possible to influence the activity of our body's chemical plant in a positive way, I set out to find more specific information.

To get started, I read a trove of international scientific articles. In general, reading broadly helps you to put specific topics in context, and I recommend it also in this case. Beyond the scientific background, I decided to look for some real-life experience. I wanted to talk to people who had experimented with solutions. I live in Israel, so I started to look for information close to me. I found a website (http://sukeret.net/) dealing with the subject ("sukeret" means diabetes in Hebrew and, unfortunately, the website is in Hebrew only). The website is run by Elan Oz, who self-cured himself of type 2 diabetes and decided to help others do the same. The large number of verifiable video testimonials by actual individuals found on the website impressed me, so I made an appointment to see him. As is always my policy when learning new areas, I approached the meeting armed with a healthy measure of skepticism. I liked what I saw when I met him, particularly the fact that he didn't try to sell me miraculous cures or potions, and that he showed me real and convincing medical records, pretty much like I am doing here now for you. I decided to go ahead and see what I could learn from him.

Elan gave me suggestions, tips, and continued support for a couple of months, until I felt that I knew where I was going and no longer needed it. He didn't sell me any snake oil, empty promises, or fake assurances; he walked me through his suggestions and shared his experience with me, he let me see his medical records showing results that one can't argue with (like my own that I am giving you here) and left the rest to me. He deserves great credit for making me believe that a cure is possible, because without that belief I wouldn't have done all it takes to succeed.

I now know what it takes to reach healthy glucose levels without having to swallow drugs every day and, in all honesty, I must caution you that it isn't an easy task. You need to be determined to achieve that result and if you start your voyage along that road, you'll encounter crises and will be tempted to give up and start taking those pills again. After all (you'll ask yourself when you are disheartened by some less-than-encouraging glucose reading), why is that such a big deal? You swallow them and your blood glucose level stays where the medical profession tells you that it should be, so why not? But you know that you should only do that if you have no other choice. And if you are strong-willed, a time will come very soon (3–4 months) when you will refuse to go back to the old ways. The best part is that you will start to reap benefits immediately and to feel better than you have ever felt in recent memory.

My Roadmap

I went through three stages: 1) priming my body prior to stop taking medicines; 2) changing my body's habits and, more importantly, my attitude toward a number of things; and 3) moving to a maintenance mode where some of the more stringent rules I had set for myself could be relaxed. In the chapters to follow I will describe those three stages in detail.

I can't stress enough that this book is only about my personal experience and was written to share with you the results I have accomplished and the journey on which I have embarked to get there. I am not a qualified health professional, and I don't presume to prescribe a cure. I am someone just like you, with no extraordinary abilities, but with a determination not to let Life push me around without fighting back. I'll say it again: this book is only about my personal experience. Before you decide to follow in my footsteps you should consult your physician and bring him or her on board, to work alongside you in this endeavor. If your doctor is a reasonable person and is willing to expend the mental effort needed to listen to you, and if you provide the reasonable arguments, questions, and considerations that this book will supply to you, there is no reason why your doctor won't work with you. I did it solo, because I didn't have any facts to show my doctor, but that's not the responsible thing to do, if you can help it.

Finally, although I have heard about a very high success rate among people who have followed Elan Oz's route, obviously there will always be cases that cannot be cured in that way and people who need to continue taking medication. However, even they can benefit from a reduction in the dose of drug that they have to take and from the improvement in the general health of their body. Still, diabetes can be a life-threatening condition and the more severe the initial condition, the more important it is to stay under proper medical supervision at all times.

The protocol that I will outline in the following chapters has worked very well for me, but that does not mean that it will work at all for you, and it may have different effects on you than it had on me, because every person is unique (as I will discuss more in later chapters). You must be your own planner and find the best route for you. Please use the information in this book responsibly and apply a grain of salt to everything you decide to do. And when (not if) you are successful, please drop me a line.

CHAPTER 2
Why We Are Unique

Before we delve into the actual process, plan, and practical stages of beating type 2 diabetes mellitus (also known in medical literature as T2DM and from now on nicknamed T2D), we must understand some basic concepts and truths. The first fact is that modern medicine is at the same time a tremendous success, and an utter failure. There is no denying that medical science has brought us almost magic treatments that save lives and improve the quality of life for entire populations that only a few decades ago were left untreated. My great aunt died of tuberculosis because antibiotics had not yet been invented, and my uncle died of a heart attack because at the time coronary bypasses were still considered an experimental procedure. The solution to those and many other illnesses have been largely found, but, on the way to producing those results, our individuality has been lost. We have become part of a range of statistics.

Human and mice both share about 97.5% of total working DNA (some articles give slightly different figures, but we won't split hairs here) and yet, we are so different. Rats live three years and we live (hopefully) 80–100 years. Those huge differences come from a mere 2.5% difference in DNA.

Humans, in contrast, differ from one another in about 1% of the DNA. That may seem a small difference, but it is in fact huge in many senses. For instance, recent studies have shown that dietary advice is largely nonsensical, because some people will gain weight with the same diet that works wonders on others,[3] and the reason is that we are different. Each one of us is unique and reacts differently to different stimuli, be they foods or drugs. But that doesn't stop modern medicine from classifying us. If you are a male, over 50, and have condition X, you need the blue pill, and if you are a woman over 65 who has osteoporosis, you need the pink one. But two men over 50 with the same condition will react differently to their pill, and so will two osteoporotic women over 65.

A paper[4] published by scientists at the Weizmann Institute recently highlighted these differences. It demonstrated statistically significant interpersonal variability in the glycemic response to different bread types, suggesting that the lack of phenotypic difference between the bread types stems from a person-specific effect—or translated into understandable, simple English: each person reacts individually to the type of bread. It further concluded that a crossover trial shows no differential clinical effect of white versus sourdough bread and that the glycemic response to the two types of bread varies greatly across people. So, when the various health authorities and organizations tell you that whole grain is good for your health and is better for you than something else if your blood sugar level is elevated, they don't know what they are talking about. It is understandable that they feel a need to say something, to give some guidance. However, instead of stating nonsense, they would do better simply by telling you that

---

[3] https://www.nytimes.com/2016/12/12/health/weight-loss-obesity.html?mcubz=2
[4] http://www.cell.com/cell-metabolism/abstract/S1550-4131(17)30288-7

which kind of food is good for you cannot be predicted, and that you should learn it on your own. Oh, but then that wouldn't be *real* guidance, would it? It would undermine their authority, wouldn't it?

Once upon a time, there was a thing called "bedside manner." I still remember our family physician, who, when I was a little boy, used to come to our house when I was sick. He always sat with me on my bed, asked questions, and then sat with my parents for a cup of coffee. I felt that he *knew* me and I trusted him to give me the medicine I needed. When he said that whatever illness I had would pass in a couple of days, I felt better already because I knew that he had followed me since I was a baby and knew how I would respond to his treatment or to my mother's chicken soup. But those days are past and gone. Today's physicians must treat so many people in so little time that they simply cannot get to know you. And then, they have the cursed thing called "protocol," which they must follow, or they may be accused of malpractice.

The other curse of modern medicine is specialization. If your little finger hurts, you must go and see a Little Finger Specialist to whom your general practitioner will refer you. He knows everything about little fingers, but he doesn't know you. To him you are not a person with all the complexity that it involves, you are a "hurting little finger case" to be treated according to protocol.

That's why when my blood sugar went skyrocketing my doctor immediately prescribed blue pills, which she tooted as the best and most modern solution to my T2D. She didn't sit with me and suggest that I should try first to lower my blood sugar through exercise and a diet. She didn't say, "try this and try that and then come to me to report on the progress that you are making." She didn't ask me if I was stressed, what I was eating, and, in general, what was going on with me (see

Chapter 5). She didn't think about it, not because she is a bad doctor—in fact, she is a great doctor in comparison to many others that I have known. However, they never trained her to do what it takes to guide me through my plight. She is conditioned to work exactly as the system requires of her and she doesn't have the time, knowledge, or freedom to work outside the very specific guidelines that someone who doesn't know me from Adam has drafted for a case like mine. That's because when you get sick, to modern medicine you are "a case," not a person.

You are on your own

All that means that as far as "unconventional" treatment is concerned (meaning a treatment that is not the standard one your doctor finds in the book), you are on your own. Once you realize that, you also understand that you must take control of your life and make decisions that you would prefer to leave to your physician, because he or she is supposed to know a lot more than you do. In reality, it is the joint knowledge of your doctor and yourself that is the right combination. You know much more about your body than you actually realize (I'll expand on that in Chapter 5), and you must trust yourself. If you feel that your body is telling you something that clashes with what you are doing or with what your doctor wants you to do, listen to it and discuss it with your doctor. Be insistent; don't let your doctor brush it away as "non-scientific nonsense."

In the introduction to this book I promised to share the results of my tests with you, and this is where I can exemplify this point with actual data that show why blindly following your doctor's prescription may be a fatal mistake. Figure 3 below is a screenshot of the readings of my albumin/creatinine ratio at the relevant testing dates (indicated beside each result—again in the DD/MM/YY format).

**Fig. 3: Albumin/Creatinine Ratio Readings.
Source: Kfir's Maccabi Healthcare Online Records**

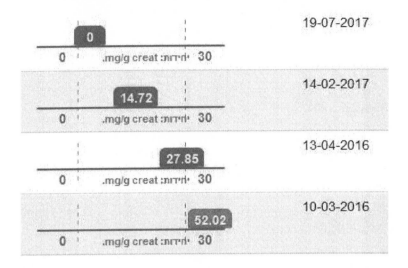

If you are not familiar with this ratio, what it means is that if you have a reading above 30 mg/g, you have a hidden kidney disease that, if left untreated, will destroy your kidneys. That is typical of diabetics. My reading on March 10, 2016 was 52.02 mg/g, so my doctor dutifully prescribed a drug that I would take for the rest of my life. Based on what the medical literature says, her prescription was entirely reasonable and to the point. But, again, the medical literature was not developed by studying Kfir's kidneys—it is based on statistical data of a large number of non-Kfir individuals.

I read about the drug and its side effects, and taking it didn't feel right to me. For whatever reason (for now call it intuition, but we will discuss it more later), I felt that I had to give my kidneys a chance before I became drug-dependent. My doctor was unhappy, but grudgingly agreed to wait one month (but no more!) and to delay treatment until the next test would convince me that I was being capricious. The next reading was high, but inside the norm, and the last reading was zero!

Had I followed my doctor's well-meaning instructions I would be taking a drug that I don't need, which has undesirable side effects, some of them quite unpleasant in the long term. This doesn't mean that my doctor's suggestions are usually wrong. On the contrary, they are usually perfectly right. I want to make it clear that I'm not suggesting that you should ignore your doctor's advice or stop taking your medicine without appropriate precautions. What I am suggesting is that you should be in command of your health, question each and every conclusion and recommendation that the medical system gives you, and test your unique body's reaction, within safe and responsible limits, to achieve the best health that you can get and deserve.

Having made all the above clear and understanding that your doctor's precepts are not to be considered a Bible to be followed blindly, let's now move on to beating T2D!

CHAPTER 3
The Three Stages

As I said before, I recognize three main stages to the process of getting in command of your blood sugar level, which I will discuss below in more detail. Before we get to it, however, I need to say a few words about monitoring your blood glucose. In the initial stages, you will have to monitor it continuously and that means pricking your finger every day and, at times, more than once a day. That cannot be avoided, not only because you must remain aware of your situation and take immediate measures if the glucose level goes too high or too low, but also because it is the only way in which you can really learn your body's preference for foods and food combinations, which is critical data.

Another important parameter is your body weight. If you have T2D it is very likely that you are overweight (which I will discuss in greater detail in Chapter 6). In Tables 1–3 below you will see my weight readings appearing sporadically beside the glucose readings. That weight data is meaningful, as you will appreciate later on.

In the following chapters, I will go into the details of what I did during the three stages to which I refer, but for now I will give you an overview and the actual raw data, so you can better appreciate my explanations going forward.

Priming Stage
In the priming stage, I wanted to get my body ready to give up medication, but I continued to take my medicine as usual. The table below shows my readings during the priming period (the dates are in the DD/MM/YY format). All glucose readings were taken using an Accu-Check© Performa Nano glucometer.

Table 1: Priming Stage Readings

Date	Morning	Evening	Weight (Kg.)
27.3.17		118	
28.3.17	134	123	82.2
29.3.17	123	109	
30.3.17	116	119	
31.3.17	116	108	
1.4.17	117	125	
2.4.17	114	108	81.3
3.4.17	109	111	
4.4.17	98	95	

Morning readings refer to fasting levels taken immediately after awakening, and I took evening readings immediately before dinner. I tried to have dinner always at the same hour (but Life got in the way, some of the time). Note that I continued to take my medicine throughout the priming period. In view of the continuous lowering of my glucose levels, I decided on April 4 to stop taking drugs. This priming stage only took me eight days, but of course, it would have taken longer if the glucose level were slower to drop.

You don't need to put a deadline to it. When your blood sugar goes down below 100 you must be vigilant not to go into hypoglycemia and, therefore, it is time to stop taking your usual drug. However, in the days immediately after discontinuing treatment, you must monitor your blood sugar level very closely and, if for whatever reason it bounces back to a high level, you must take your medicine again and consult with your doctor.

Habits-changing Stage
Old habits die hard, but as I will explain, doing a complete revision of your habits is a critical factor for a successful result. That's why this was a much longer stage than the priming one, taking about one month. On April 5, I stopped taking my medicine, and the reading on April 6 is the first drug-free one.

Table 2: Habits-changing Stage Readings

Date	Morning	Evening	Weight (Kg.)
6.4.17	116	109	
7.4.17	110	95	
8.4.17	113	100	
9.4.17	111	87	
10.4.17	119	104	
11.4.17	106	89	81
12.4.17	107	95	
13.4.17	123	113	
14.4.17	129	94	
15.4.17	111	93	

Table 2: Continued			
16.4.17	108	86	79.8
17.4.17	115	82	
18.4.17	118	88	
19.4.17	102	92	
20.4.17	110	89	
21.4.17	121	78	
22.4.17	109	97	79.2
23.4.17	119	93	
24.4.17	109	96	
25.4.17	124	84	78.9
26.4.17	105	87	
27.4.17	121	97	
28.4.17	107	83	
29.4.17	109	118	78.7
30.4.17	109	94	
1.5.17	115	95	
2.5.17	116	101	
3.5.17	117	91	
4.5.17	105	95	
5.5.17	119	98	78.2
6.5.17	111	102	
7.5.17	110	97	
8.5.17	103	92	

Note that glucose levels are quite low in the evening, in spite of the proper breakfast, lunch, and snacks I had during the day.

Maintenance Mode Stage

The maintenance mode is, essentially, what my new life looks like. At the time of releasing this book, my fasting blood glucose bounces around 100 ± 10 and gets me the normal HbA1C that I need. I expect this value to improve further with time, but that may be a slow process evolving over the next few months. When that happens significantly, I will post the results on my website (www.doitwithwords.com) to keep readers informed.

Table 3: Maintenance Mode Stage Readings

Date	Morning	Evening	Weight (Kg.)
9.5.17	111		
10.5.17	119		
11.5.17	111		
12.5.17	119		77.7
13.5.17	112		
14.5.17	114		
15.5.17	117		
16.5.17	120		
17.5.17	110		
18.5.17	110		77.1
19.5.17	105		
20.5.17	102		
21.5.17	112		
22.5.18	105		

Table 3: Continued			
23.5.17	111		
24.5.17	118		
25.5.17	124		
26.5.17	95		
27.5.17	105		
28.5.17	--		76.8
29.5.18	111		
30.5.18	100		
31.5.17	109		
1.6.17	106		
2.6.17	120		
3.6.17	104		76.5
4.6.17	105		
5.6.17	117		
10.6.17	120		75.5
16.6.17	123		75.5
18.6.17	111		
19.6.17	104		
5.7.17	--		76.5
11.7.17	117		76.1
18.7.17	113		
19.7.17	102		

Since checking my levels every day had become somewhat boring and unnecessary, in view of the essentially constant results I got, at the beginning of June I decided to switch to testing every few days and also, confident as I was in what I was doing, I took a vacation from it (coinciding with my actual summer vacation). I now test my glucose levels once a week in the morning.

The process combines a number of different activities that are its building blocks and before we can put them to a useful purpose, we must understand them, their role, and their importance. That is what we will do in the coming chapters.

CHAPTER 4
Eating Right

Eating the right food is the cornerstone of your effort. As I said before, your body is a complex chemical plant in which many different processes run in parallel, and a change that you make to the "raw material" that you feed to your plant may influence a number of them and, as a result, the chemistry of your body. Based on what we have learned today from new research (see Chapter 2), I believe that dietary advice is useless and may even be deleterious. Telling you to eat two types of food together (or not to eat them together) may work well for one person and may be a disaster for another. Following complicated diets is often not really rewarding and a substantial hassle, so after a while you stop following them and that may be all for the best. The only person who seems to benefit from the complex, convoluted, and at times sadistic dietary instructions appears to be your dietician, or at least their bank account.

My take on dieting is very simple: eat everything except forbidden foods. When you look at the list of forbidden foods, at first you may think that you are left with nothing to eat, but soon you will see that, on the contrary, you can eat many diverse foods and you can discover the joy of wholesome dishes that you have ignored for years. You will also discover that counting calories is no longer that important, and that you are never to be hungry again (in contrast to what happens when you take up the fancy diet of the moment). Without further ado, let's start talking about forbidden and recommended foods.

Further on in this chapter I will give examples of what I eat and have eaten during the three stages, but this is not a recipe book. You will find that recipes for meals based on the foods recommended below are readily available (but you will be able to make your own choices quite simply without having to study them). One of the things I have learned is that, to succeed in keeping a healthy eating regimen, it has to be simple and it should not require you to worry all the time about what you will eat next.

FORBIDDEN FOODS
Wheat
The first and greatest enemy of your blood sugar level is wheat in all its forms. This is also the biggest sacrifice that you must make—giving up wheat in all its forms. No more bread, cookies with coffee, and the myriad of tasty, warm, and sugary wheat products that call to us from every shelf. The moment you decide to start working on your T2D you must resolve to give up wheat, and that's not negotiable. To me, a born Italian, giving up spaghetti and 1000 other delicious pasta dishes felt like the end of the world, but the good news is that after a short while you stop craving wheat. As I said, continuing to eat wheat products is not an option, so if you decide that you can't live without them, stop reading now. Giving up wheat is a bit like quitting smoking (I know because I've done both) and is really the hardest part of this program.

There are two good reasons for not eating wheat products: First, it is the most invasive carb around, found almost everywhere, and carbs translate in your body immediately into sugar. But then, and perhaps even more importantly, wheat contains gluten. A short while ago I ran into Dr. William Davis' excellent book, *Wheat Belly*, in which he explains, on the basis of sound scientific evidence, why modern wheat, which has been genetically modified, is particularly harmful to our health. I wish I had read Dr. Davis' book before I embarked on my program, because it would have made it so much easier for me to renounce wheat. Reading it and seeing the implications of his data scared the hell out of me, and I will never crave bread or pasta again. For that reason, I recommend reading *Wheat Belly*, as a motivational aid in giving up wheat altogether, and because it has a wealth of information on what you should and shouldn't eat, including many interesting recipes. I had to learn how to prepare tasty, wheat-free dishes for myself. You don't have to.

Staying clear of wheat products has another extremely important effect: it makes you lose weight. I eat a lot and much of what I eat is caloric (for instance, cheese like Cheddar or Swiss) and I lose weight without effort. Don't be confused by my weight readings in Table 3, which show an increase of 0.5–1 Kg (1.1–2.2 pounds)—which is due to increased muscle mass that I will discuss in Chapter 6.

Divorcing wheat is for good and you must make peace with that. That doesn't mean that, in time, you won't be able to eat half a biscuit with tea, but that's pretty much as far as you can plan to go.

Carbohydrates

You must adopt a carbs-free diet, because carbs wind up as sugar in your bloodstream. However, your diet will never be really carbs-free, because carbs hide everywhere and you will be getting some no matter what you eat. That's a good thing, because, to be balanced, your diet needs to supply *some* carbs to your body. However, according to Dr. Davis, if you want to undo diabetes you must keep your carbs intake at less than 30 gr per day.

Moreover, while in the first two stages you need to adopt a religiously strict avoidance of carbs; in the maintenance stage, after you reach your goal, you will be able to slacken those rules a bit and eat *some* carbs, sometimes. (Please also see Chapter 9 for a discussion on slackening rules and suggestions for doing so.)

You may not always know what contains carbs and what doesn't. Carbs, as I said, hide in unexpected places and so you should rely on glycemic index tables published by serious sources, such as that published by the Harvard Medical School.[5] You may of course already be familiar with these tables, if you've been coping with T2D for a while, but perhaps you didn't think of it as a tool to discover hidden carbs. The table will tell you if a food that you are planning to eat has a high glycemic index (in which case you don't want to eat it anyway), but be aware that it may also give you tantalizingly low values for wheat products, which doesn't mean that you are allowed to eat them (for instance, the index for fettuccini is only 32, but wheat is wheat).

Anything with sugar in it

I know that our mothers wanted us to eat fruit because it is healthy, but fruit is full of sugar so it is not allowed at all in the first two stages. Sure, you need vitamins, but please go and get them from veggies. However, some fruit is less sugary than others (berries, apples), and in the third stage you will be able to eat them every now and then, provided you test yourself for each variety and make sure that it doesn't unexpectedly shoot your blood sugar sky-high (again, we are unique also in that each individual reacts differently to the same food, and a reputedly safe food may not be that good for you).

My personal peeve is that I can't eat chocolate. I love

---

[5] http://www.health.harvard.edu/diseases-and-conditions/glycemic-index-and-glycemic-load-for-100-foods

chocolate and I must make do with second-best brands, sweetened with stevia (the only sweetener that you should use, and even that only on occasions). I've come to terms with that.

Alcohol
Sorry, no booze. That is one of the biggest no-nos. However, if you are a wine lover like myself, you can look forward to drinking a half glass of red wine at lunch, starting with the third stage.

Artificial Sweeteners
Anything with artificial sweeteners in it must be off the table. That includes sodas and all the so-called "dietary products." It takes about two weeks to get used to drinking unsweetened coffee and tea, and the big bonus is that after you clean your taste buds of those chemicals your food starts to taste much better. Believe me, you have nothing to lose by not sweetening your drinks. And I've discovered that I can enjoy my meal with water or soda water just as well.

Beer
That's another one that got me sighing, but there's nothing I can do—stay away from beer. Besides, the alcohol, it has other undesirable ingredients in it. A basic component of beer is a starch source, such as malted barley, which is able to be saccharified (converted to sugars) then fermented (converted into ethanol and carbon dioxide). That's poison to you. You should note that the reason beer is not mentioned in the glycemic index tables is not that it is glycemically safe, but rather that beer's glycemic index cannot be tested due to its low carbohydrate content. However, "low" here means "low for measuring purposes," not for your blood sugar. For example, a 300ml beer will have around 10g of carbohydrate, which is a third of your total permissible daily intake. Drinking beer will

increase blood glucose levels, whether it is in the glycemic index table or not.

Processed Food

Processed food is bad for you, period. Don't be tempted to believe the labels and the ads that tell you how healthy morning cereals are, or how well-looked-after were the pigs that went into your hot dog. Particularly, avoid all the so-called "gluten-free" products. As Dr. Davis explains, many gluten-free foods are made by replacing wheat flour with cornstarch, rice starch, potato starch, or tapioca starch (starch extracted from the root of the cassava plant). This is especially hazardous for anybody looking to drop twenty, thirty, or more pounds, since gluten-free foods, though they do not trigger the immune or neurological response of wheat gluten, still trigger the glucose-insulin response that causes you to gain weight. Wheat products increase blood sugar and insulin more than most other foods, but foods made with cornstarch, rice starch, potato starch, and tapioca starch are among the few foods that increase blood sugar even more than wheat products.

Many ready-to-use salad dressings also contain thickeners and flavors that are starchy and bad for you. Similarly, ketchup often contains sucrose or high-fructose corn syrup. I only use lemon, vinegar (preferably apple vinegar), and, occasionally, balsamic vinegar, together with olive oil, to dress my salad, and I recommend them for great taste.

RECOMMENDED FOODS

So, is there anything left to eat? Plenty.

Vegetables

With few exceptions, eat vegetables as much and as frequently as you wish. The exceptions include peas, carrots, potatoes, chickpeas, lentils, and tomatoes (I love tomatoes, but the sugar content is too high).

Meat

Unprocessed meat is fine. Of course, if you have a very high cholesterol or uric acid problem, you should avoid red meat as much as possible and eat more poultry instead. However, I have found that eating meat at dinner may adversely affect my morning levels. Again, that's only me and it may be that you won't experience any difference when eating meat. However, taking into account that getting a good night's sleep is also extremely important (see Chapter 7), eating lightly at night is better. Vegetables and fish are always a good choice for dinner.

Fish

I have always loved fish, and I love it more now that I have discovered more varieties and cooking styles, simply by paying more attention to what I'm going to eat. I'm less happy about shellfish, and I eat it only very sparingly, if at all. For whatever reason, with my current diet it doesn't seem as tasty as it used to. When you change your diet as drastically as I have done, your taste changes, mostly for the better.

Smoked salmon is great for breakfast, together with cheese or fried eggs, and so is tuna.

Dairy Products

Dairy products are okay, but milk contains sugar so it should be consumed in small amounts. Hard and aged cheese is particularly good for a snack.

Nuts

Nuts are my favorite snack and I always keep a bag of mixed nuts with me. Dr. T. Colin Campbell praises the many benefits of eating nuts.[6] All I can add is that they are tasty as well.

Eggs
Eggs are an important component of my diet, particularly in the morning and after I exercise.

Green Tea
Green tea is considered to have a host of beneficial effects,[7] although not all studies agree on them and possibly not all mentioned advantages are real or substantial. Among the benefits relevant to this discussion, you will find:

1. Green tea increases fat burning and improves physical performance. Green tea has been shown to increase fat burning and boost the metabolic rate in human-controlled trials, although not all studies agree.

2. Green tea may lower your risk of type 2 diabetes (and, arguably, help to control it). Some controlled trials show that green tea can cause mild reductions in blood sugar levels.

3. Green tea can help you lose weight and lower your risk of becoming obese. Some studies show that green tea leads to increased weight loss. It is particularly effective at reducing dangerous abdominal fat.

4. It is delicious. So many varieties of green tea exist on the market that everybody can find the varieties they like.

However, if you drink a lot of tea, as well as water, and particularly if you exercise intensively, make sure to add sufficient amounts of salt to your diet, particularly if you are on a low sodium diet, because drinking a lot and sweating may make you lose too much sodium, which may be dangerous.

---

[6] https://bluezones.com/2017/07/why-nuts-are-nutritional-powerhouse
[7] https://authoritynutrition.com/top-10-evidence-based-health-benefits-of-green-tea

AN EXEMPLARY DAY

The first thing to keep in mind is that, to be successful, you must make breakfast your main meal. There are many different reasons for this, practical and philosophical, but the reality (based on my experience) is that dinner should be skimpy, while lunch should be mostly veggies. But if you play your cards right, you won't be hungry. An important trick for the first stage and at least half of the second, is to remember to eat something between meals, every three–four hours. In time, your hunger will diminish and you'll be satisfied with a light snack, every now and then.

So here's how I did it:

Morning

A large salad with olive oil and lemon dressing, or olive oil and apple vinegar dressing. One or two scrambled eggs or half a portion of tuna in oil or water, or sliced smoked salmon. Sometimes I add a bit of cream or cottage cheese or something similar. A cup of unsweetened coffee or green tea goes with that.

Until Lunch

Nowadays I don't do it much anymore, but until your stomach shrinks I recommend bringing with you to work a box with raw cucumbers and bell peppers (except the green ones, which may actually be immature, non-ripe versions of other color varieties and may have lower contents of healthy vitamin C and carotenoids), and any other vegetable you fancy, cut into strips, and to eat as much as you want of them, but without forgetting to eat something at least four hours after breakfast. You must not be hungry because hunger may cause your blood glucose to plummet, which may be dangerous. If you feel empty, eat these.

When, after a period of time, you feel only a little empty in

KFIR LUZZATTO

between meals, I recommend eating a few assorted nuts with a cup of tea. Generally speaking, drink as much green tea as you can between meals. The only disadvantage to drinking green tea is the need to visit the restroom more often, but it helps while away the time until the next meal.

Lunch

What to eat at lunch depends very much on what you had at breakfast, because you don't want to get bored. The basis should again be a salad, but if you had eggs for breakfast you may want to make a tuna salad. Conversely, if you had tuna in the morning, you may want to bring a hardboiled egg with you to add to your salad. Another good option is hard cheese to go with it. There is no limit to the amount of vegetables that you can eat, but you need to go slow on the fats and proteins. Adding avocado to your salad is in many cases quite satisfying, as is adding pumpkin or sunflower seeds to it. These are only examples and you can and should be creative with it.

If you work away from home, I strongly suggest that you take lunch with you. I find that preparing the exact lunch that you want by yourself is truly satisfying (please don't let your significant other do it, and also read on this respect in Chapter 9). You know exactly what to expect and you don't eat wrong food because you are in a hurry or because you can't find the right things where you are eating. It is important.

I know, as a grown-up person you may be embarrassed at first, taking a lunchbox with you like you did in kindergarten. Get over it. After you do it a few times you'll wonder why you never did it before.

Between Lunch and Dinner

I find that a snack consisting of a 3% yoghurt and a handful of assorted nuts gets me through the day and to dinner with a

. 32 .

healthy appetite, without being famished. But again, as long as you don't stray from the basic rules of no carbs and mostly vegetables, you are fine. Semi-hard cheese with nuts also works well for me as a snack, mostly on weekends when I have the opportunity to pick from a selection of cheese in my fridge.

Dinner

Dinner should be the lightest possible, preferably without protein. But if you crave some protein, a small fish fillet is probably the best choice. I very much enjoy having grilled vegetables, lightly seasoned with olive oil and balsamic vinegar. I find that a plate including eggplant, bell pepper, onion, and zucchini, is most satisfying. If you prefer your vegetables sautéed, additional options include broccoli, asparagus, Brussels sprouts, and cabbage. There is a whole world out there, waiting for you to discover, and a wealth of veggie recipes everywhere you turn, online and in books.

I am not trying to give you detailed instructions to follow day by day. That's exactly what made all the diets I tried before fail miserably. You don't need it, once you understand the basic blueprint of what you should and should not do, which is easily derivable from the example given above. If you need more examples of daily menus, I again recommend looking at the recipes in Dr. Davis' book. But in the end you need to see what works for you, for your own body's chemical plant. Don't let anybody tell you what's good for you, particularly not the purveyors of fake, fashionable diets. You are perfectly capable of deciding for yourself what foods you like and how they influence your body.

CHAPTER 5
It's All in Your Brain

Before we move on to the additional practical steps that you should take to fight your T2D, besides eating right, it is important to understand the role that our mind plays in all this. I am firmly convinced that the key to success in all practices that require strength of character and determination, is a complete and unreserved belief in the possibility that you may succeed in reaching your goal. I say "possibility," not "certainty," because you may fail even if you should be able to succeed, and even when you are attempting something that anybody else can do. That may happen simply because you got some detail wrong, or because of some innate difference between you and the rest of the world. I can't offer any mathematical proof of the truth of these precepts, and you must reach your own conviction that I am right, through your own experience. I can only relate to you what I know to be true for me and that I believe to be a universal truth.

Have you ever thought how is it that your body is capable of running a myriad of complex biochemical reactions all the time, and getting everything running smoothly and correctly? Who is sitting in the control room of your "chemical factory" and making sure that everything is timed right? All those processes run autonomously, without the need for your intervention, because if they needed you to run them, you would die right away. But although your mind doesn't need you to run the show, you may influence its activity and steer it in a desired direction, at least to some extent.

A discussion of the many ways in which you can influence what your mind does to your body is outside the scope of this book. However, there is at least one topic that must be discussed, and that is stress. Stress has been known since the seventeenth century to be a potential contributor to chronic hyperglycemia in diabetes.[8] Nevertheless, when you went to your doctor to talk about your T2D, did he or she tell you that the first thing that you should do is take control of, and drastically reduce, your stress level? No? I thought so.

As Dr. Scott M. Fried explains well in his book *A Surgeon's Self-Hypnosis Healing Solution*,[9] most disease processes, like nerve injury, heart disease, high blood pressure, adult onset diabetes, osteoarthritis, and many cancers, develop slowly through cumulative micro traumas to our bodies. These small, often self-induced miniature traumas, when recognized, can be stopped or mitigated and the long- term effects avoided. And we can reverse these disease processes simply by relaxing, changing behavior patterns, slowing down, and regenerating in a proper way. You didn't know that, did you? And how could you, if your doctor didn't tell you?

If I can't convince you to invest in relaxing and reducing your stress levels and by that improving your glucose blood level, there is little I can convince you to do. It doesn't cost you anything, it makes you feel great, and improves your health, so

---

[8] Richard S. Surwit, PhD, Mark S. Schneider, PhD and Mark N. Feinglos, MD, *"Stress in Diabetes Mellitus,"* *Diabetes Care 1992 Oct; 15*(10): 1413–1422. *https://doi.org/10.2337/diacare.15.10.1413*
[9] Fried, Dr. Scott M., *A Surgeon's Self-Hypnosis Healing Solution – My Father's Secret.* Kindle Edition

please take it seriously. There are many ways to reduce stress and you must pick the one or two that are best for you. Some of it will be achieved through physical exercise, which is a necessity that will be covered in Chapter 6. Other ways include self-hypnosis, guided imagery, and taking your spouse to the movies more frequently. If you choose to investigate those options, I can recommend the following references, all which are readily available from Amazon's Kindle shop:

1. ***Guided Imagery for Self-Healing,*** by Martin L. Rossman, M.D.

2. ***More Instant Self-Hypnosis: Hypnotize Yourself as You Read,*** by Forbes Robbins Blair.

3. ***Change Your Life with Self-Hypnosis,*** by Michael Hadfield.

I have said it before and I'll say it again, not to discourage you but, on the contrary, to encourage you. What you want to accomplish is not an easy task and you need to convince yourself that the prize is worth the effort. It is. By starting to invest in this process you will see results pretty soon and that will cement your belief. There is nothing more convincing than doing things designed to lower your blood sugar, and actually finding in the morning that it is the lowest you have seen in a long time. The reason why you need faith in your ability to succeed is that, sometimes your reading will be higher after a few days in which you saw improvement, and you may feel discomfited. But we are not machines and we have ups and downs. That's human. You may have done everything right, eaten right, exercised right, and still your reading may be higher than it was yesterday. When that happens, think back over your day: Was it a hard day at the office, did you get excited about anything, do you feel stressed out, did you omit to relax a bit when you came home yesterday, did you eat a new variety of food? Or maybe you did all you can, and your reading is inexplicably high. That happens and it is okay. You can't let a little setback discourage you. You're better than that!

Listen to Your Body

As I hinted before, you know much more about your body than you realize you do. Dr. Martin Rossman[10] explains that "intuition is defined as 'power of knowing without recourse to reason' and is perceived by inner seeing, inner listening, and inner feeling. It may well be a specialized function of the right hemisphere of the brain. Through the right brain's ability to perceive subtle cues regarding feelings and connections, we are guided by what we call instincts, gut feelings, and hunches. By becoming quiet and attentive to our inner thoughts, we can use the talents of this neglected part of our minds most effectively."

You must listen to your body because although it will never send you a detailed memo, it continuously signals to you important information about what is happening in your "chemical plant." If you choose to ignore its signals, you are missing out on what could be the most important data needed to achieve wellbeing. I have learned to listen to my body and to pay attention to what it is telling me, and I never discount intuitive thoughts about my health. The example that I gave in Chapter 2 illustrates this point very well. I didn't know why my doctor's diagnosis didn't sound right to me, but the feeling was clear enough for me to question the wisdom of starting treatment without an in-depth check, regardless of how hard my doctor worked to scare me into beginning immediately to swallow chemicals. Once again, this book is not meant to discuss the topic of the mind–body connection in detail. Many good

---

[10] Rossman, Martin L., *Guided Imagery for Self-Healing: An Essential Resource for Anyone Seeking Wellness* (Kindle Locations 1597–1601). New World Library. Kindle Edition.

references exist on the subject, but the important point is to recognize that our mind has an influence on how our body treats glucose levels, because it is our mind that manages our body's chemical plant. Accordingly, we must not neglect our mental wellbeing, and particularly stress, when we seek to overcome T2D.

This is well expressed by the American Diabetes Association:[11]

"Stress results when something causes your body to behave as if it were under attack. Sources of stress can be physical, like injury or illness. Or they can be mental, like problems in your marriage, job, health, or finances.

"When stress occurs, the body prepares to take action. This preparation is called the fight-or-flight response. In the fight-or-flight response, levels of many hormones shoot up. Their net effect is to make a lot of stored energy—glucose and fat—available to cells. These cells are then primed to help the body get away from danger.

"In people who have diabetes, the fight-or-flight response does not work well. Insulin is not always able to let the extra energy into the cells, so glucose piles up in the blood."

But reducing stress may be easier said than done, if you are under an objectively stressing situation, like illness in the family, demanding work, etc. Still, there are things you can do to reduce stress levels. One particularly enjoyable option, if you can make the time, is practicing yoga. In a 2014 study[12] (Effects of Yogic Exercises on Life Stress and Blood Glucose Levels in Nursing Students), the author found that doing yogic exercises for 60 minutes one day a week for 12 weeks, including physical exercise combined with relaxation and meditation, significantly decreased

---

[11] http://www.diabetes.org/living-with-diabetes/complications/mental-health/stress.html

[12] https://www.ncbi.nlm.nih.gov/pmc/articles/PMC4273078/

both stress and postprandial blood glucose levels compared with the control group (which did not exercise).

Other options for reducing stress include guided imagery and self-hypnosis, but you really need to find out what works for you. The main thing is to do *something* to reduce your stress level. If a walk in the park does it for you, that's great, and so it is if listening to classical music works as a stress killer for you.

And then, of course, there is physical exercise, discussed in the next chapter.

CHAPTER 6
Exercise

If you hate going to the gym, this book is not for you. The American Diabetes Association[13] advocates exercise because "there are a few ways that exercise lowers blood glucose:

Insulin sensitivity is increased, so your cells are better able to use any available insulin to take up glucose during and after activity.

When your muscles contract during activity, it stimulates another mechanism that is completely separate of insulin. This mechanism allows your cells to take up glucose and use it for energy whether insulin is available or not.

"This is how exercise can help lower blood glucose in the short term. And when you are active on a regular basis, it can also lower your A1C."

Besides those advantages, exercising helps you to lose weight. Although the heavy lifting in the slimming process is done by abstaining from eating wheat products and carbs in general, exercise helps too. Moreover, exercise is important to reduce stress levels, the criticality of which was discussed in the

---

[13] http://www.diabetes.org/food-and-fitness/fitness/get-started-safely/blood-glucose-control-and-exercise.html

previous chapter.

The great thing about exercise is that it is addictive. When you exercise for a sufficient period of time you start to enjoy it and then it becomes an essential part of your day. Even if at first you struggle a bit to do it (particularly if you haven't exercised seriously for a few years), it gets easier and easier as you go.

So how much and when should you exercise? Well, the when is easy: every day. If you set it as a goal to exercise every day, even if it happens that you need to skip one day, it won't make a difference. As to how much, it is quite individual and depends on your general physical condition. You should consult with your health advisor on the kind of exercise that is healthy for you, to make sure that you are not causing any damage to your body, particularly if you have orthopedic or cardiovascular conditions. I'm over 60, so before starting to exercise seriously I took a thorough physical test to verify that my pump would be able to take it. Don't skip this step, because exercising incorrectly may have dire consequences.

Based on my experience, I suggest exercising moderately for the first three months or so. I now take a daily brisk walk (at an average speed of approximately four miles per hour or 6.5 Km/h), for 3–3.5 miles (4.8–5.5 Km), but I started out at a lower speed of about 3.8 miles/hour and distance of about 2.8 miles, building up gradually to the current values.

Depending on your physical condition, you may find as I did that after about three months cardio training ceases to be a challenge and you are no longer able to reach high heart rates (85–90% of your maximum) that burn calories and fat. Ironically, the fitter you become, the less effective your daily workout is. That may be a problem if you haven't managed to get rid of belly fat—fat in your midsection, which tends to swaddle organs that play a key role in regulating blood sugar. In and of itself, belly fat works to block the action of insulin, which is necessary to lower blood sugar—which is known as "insulin resistance."

So what to do when cardio workout is no longer as effective as at first, to reduce belly fat? If you read relevant advice on how to exercise (but be careful, please), you will find that strength training is the answer. What I have been doing, as of the middle of my maintenance stage, is to combine walking and weight lifting, the latter done for about 20 minutes three times a week on alternate days. In simplistic terms, when you lift heavy weights for a few reps, it burns all of the glycogen (sugar) stored in your muscles. When the glycogen runs out, it taps into the sugar in your blood. If you add several repetitions to your exercise, you'll burn up the muscle-stored glycogen quickly, and will keep using your muscles beyond your blood's ability to provide sugar to the muscles, so your liver will have to provide the rest of the energy. When this happens, your body has to quickly replace the glycogen that the liver has sent to the muscle. If you aren't eating immediately after the workout, there is no other source of energy for your liver than the fatty adipose tissue around your body. That extra-muscular fat will be broken down, and the fat cells will be turned into fuel to replenish the glycogen your body used. Thus, you will burn fat very effectively.

Men and women should do strength training differently, of course, because of the difference in bone and muscle structure, and before you undertake it, you should get professional advice adapted to your specific needs.

The other byproduct of strength training is an increase in muscle mass. Muscles weigh more than fat and thus you will see at this point that you are gaining weight—see for instance in Table 3 above, what happened to my weight between June 16 and July 11, 2017. My net weight gain was 600 grams (1.3 pounds), but in fact during that period I lost belly fat and the weight I gained was in my muscles. How can I tell? When you get to that point, you need to trust the old method of telling whether you are losing or gaining weight by checking your clothes. Your trousers don't lie and you can tell from them if your girth is not going in the right direction.

There is a fringe benefit to training as I do: you end up feeling great. I am full of energy and perpetually in a good mood. That is no small thing and it reflects on your health. In the past couple of months I've been rather astonished because several people whom I hadn't seen in a while felt compelled to walk up to me and tell me, "You look good," sounding honestly surprised. I can't tell you exactly what is priming these compliments—perhaps getting better inside makes you look better outside—because nothing like it has ever happened to me before, but I'm getting used to it. It's validation from people who don't know what on Earth you are doing to yourself, and is another incentive to continue on this path.

CHAPTER 7
New Habits

By now, you surely appreciate that in order to succeed you must make big changes in your lifestyle. That means, making as many radical changes as you need to implement the things you want to do. If you have been sitting down to the morning table for the past 20 years with sweet coffee and carrot cake, you can't expect to sit at the same table at the same time, with unsweetened coffee and a cold cucumber, and feel right about it. This means that you need to kill your old habits and start brand new ones that work well with your plan for getting better.

I have been a night owl all my life. I never went to bed before 1 AM and typically much later. I functioned better at night (or so I thought) and left all work that needed concentration to the small hours. Getting up in the morning has always been a torture to me and if I had to get up before 8 AM, I walked around most of the day like a zombie. When I realized that exercising for one hour or more every day was going to be a challenge, coming home late from work and feeling wasted as I was (partly because of my high blood glucose), I made a courageous decision: I would exercise in the morning. That way a long day at the office was no longer a valid excuse for skipping exercise. Now I wake up at a quarter to 6 AM, drink a cup of unsweetened coffee (and enjoy it) and go out for a walk by 6:15. If the weather does not permit it, I hit the treadmill. I go to bed by 10:30–11:00 PM and get up rested and ready in the morning. It's not my old me. I am a completely new person. Simply by making a considered decision to ditch an old habit, I have found myself in new territories where my body had no expectation of receiving familiar treatment, and I was able to put new rules in place without my mind and body feeling any sense of loss.

As a result of this radical decision I have gained much more. Another stupid habit I had was to watch the midnight news (and often to fall asleep with it or with any program that came up after it). Now I read the morning paper instead, which means that I waste only a few minutes to bring myself up to date, and I discovered that TV news is really a waste of time, which I can use to read and relax. Watching TV at night also ruins your sleep. Shawn Stevenson[14] relates that "numerous studies have confirmed that watching television before bed disrupts your sleep cycle. It might seem like a mundane activity to sit back and watch TV in your bed, but parts of your brain are being set off like fireworks. You're actually putting a stressor on your brain and body, especially if it's time to be winding down for bed." When you rewire yourself for new habits, it's a great time to revisit the old ones and to determine whether they are hurting your goal. Sleeping well is essential to being relaxed and to exercising properly, as well as to losing weight, so it is something that you need to take into account and factor in when fighting T2D.

Coming back after morning exercise and a revitalizing shower, I am more than ready for breakfast. In the past, "breakfast" to me meant mostly cereals (those that they sell to us as "healthy grain cereals" but in fact are a concentrate of

---

[14] Stevenson, Shawn. *Sleep Smarter: 21 Essential Strategies to Sleep Your Way to a Better Body, Better Health, and Bigger Success* (p. 97). Rodale Books.

harmful carbs, wheat, and non-wheat). With the exception of eggs and bacon, I never even considered eating anything at breakfast that did not have a substantial hydrocarbon component. With my eggs and bacon I always had plenty of toast with butter and jam or honey and, of course, well-sweetened coffee. Now I feast on a gorgeous salad with either tuna, smoked salmon, eggs, or cheese, washed down with unsweetened green tea, and like it!

That's the strength of habit. I'm not saying that I liked it immediately or that I thought it tastier than cereals right away. But after a while—a couple of weeks at most—I found myself enjoying it and I no longer thought of sweet breakfast foods. I had created a new habit.

I can't tell you which habits you have to lose and what parts of your day you need to turn upside-down, because I don't know you or what your day looks like. But you do, and if you are honest with yourself you know what to do and that you have no excuse for not doing it.

Don't procrastinate! You will have to give up those yummy croissants that you have been able to keep eating thanks to your glucose pills, so you may as well ditch them now.

Now, I said!

CHAPTER 8
Food Supplements

Some people will tell you that food supplements are snake oil. I agree, but nevertheless I suggest that you use them in the first two stages of your fight. I can explain that seeming contradiction in two words: placebo effect.

As Jo Marchand relates in her excellent book,[15] "placebo effects have only been studied in a few systems so far, but there are probably many others…the placebo effect isn't a single phenomenon but a 'melting pot' of responses, each using different ingredients from the brain's natural pharmacy." In other words, when we give a patient a placebo it is a cue for the brain to release materials that do the job, even though we were only given a sugar pill. But the most important effect of all, which is relevant to what we are discussing here, is the fact that placebo pills have a curative effect even when we know beforehand that they contain no drug! One of the leaders in this field of research is Harvard medical professor Ted Kaptchuk, who explained his results in a recent interview[16] that is worth reading.

---

[15] Marchant, Jo. *Cure: A Journey into the Science of Mind Over Body* (p. 17). Crown/Archetype.

[16] https://www.vox.com/science-and-health/2017/6/1/15711814/open-label-placebo-kaptchuk

This shouldn't surprise us because healing rituals have been around since the dawn of time. As said before, our brain runs the show and can tell our body's chemical factory to make chemical "products" that have a curative effect, but before it does so it must know that this is needed. A ritual—including that of taking a pill that admittedly contains no active material—appears to be a way to communicate that need to our brain. That's why I find that taking some food supplements in the first, psychologically intense stages of our fight with T2D, may have a value. Besides, I cannot rule out that some of these supplements may actually have a beneficial effect, since in some cases research exists that supports that possibility.

We shouldn't forget, however, that food supplements are chemical materials that may interact with other drugs you are taking, or may not be indicated if you have a certain condition. We have a tendency to approach natural materials differently from chemically manufactured ones, and in some cases that is right, but definitely not always. We shouldn't forget that natural drugs are still drugs. Some of the most lethal poisons are natural materials, and other seemingly innocuous products of Mother Nature can make us sick. Therefore, before you decide to take a supplement you should consult with your doctor.

Let's now run through a list of supplements that you may want to consider taking, at least until you are through with stage 2 of your work. The dose that I would consider taking is the lowest recommended in each case.

Konjac Fibers – Konjac fiber is a starch from the root of the konjac plant (Amorphophallus konjac), which grows in both China and Japan. The Japanese regard konjac as a health food, and consider it to be especially good for intestinal functioning. Its main component is glucomannan, a water-soluble dietary fiber consisting of mannose and glucose sugars. According to a

2008 review,[17] glucomannan significantly lowered total cholesterol, LDL ("bad") cholesterol, and triglycerides, kept blood sugar (glucose) stable, and had a slight effect on weight.

My own experience with konjac fibers, taken before each meal for two months, didn't lead to any disagreeable effects.

Gymnema sylvestre – Gymnema has been used to lower blood sugar, reduce the amount of sugar absorbed by the intestines, lower LDL cholesterol, and stimulate insulin release in the pancreas.

If you are anything like me, you may be struggling with a sweet tooth, which makes losing weight all the more difficult and, of course, exposes you to sugar-containing foods. Gymnema sylvestre contains gymnemic acids, which, when placed directly on your tongue, actually fill the sugar receptors in your taste buds, effectively blocking your ability to taste sweetness.[18] Whether that's a placebo effect or not, I noticed a sharp reduction in sugar craving while taking gymnema leaf capsules.

Clinical studies with gymnema sylvestre are rare (one wonders why). A human study found an insulin-elevating effect[19] as a result of gymnema's unique ability to repair beta cells in the pancreas. However, the literature mentions, besides its promise as a sugar-lowering material, also the possibility of adverse interaction with other drugs and so, before taking it, you should consult your doctor.

Korean Ginseng (root extract) – The ginseng root finds widespread recognition and has become a popular herbal remedy the world over. Its uses range from remedies for a headache,

---

[17] https://www.ncbi.nlm.nih.gov/pubmed/18842808
[18] https://www.ncbi.nlm.nih.gov/pmc/articles/PMC3912882
[19] https://www.ncbi.nlm.nih.gov/pubmed/2259217

fever, and indigestion, to the treatment of infertility and erectile dysfunction. As a stimulant, the root helps improve concentration and is used to boost memory, retention power, and general thinking. It also finds extensive use in remedies to fight depression, anxiety, and mood swings. It boosts immunity and keeps infections at bay.

However, the potentially beneficial effect that appears to be most useful in conjunction with the purposes of this book is its anti-stress action[20] (see the discussion of stress in Chapter 5).

Coenzyme Q10 – Coenzyme Q10, or CoQ10, is a substance that the human body makes naturally and cells use it to generate energy. CoQ10 is also a powerful antioxidant that helps fight free radicals that can damage cells and DNA.

As you get older, your body produces less and less CoQ10. People with diabetes and other conditions (such as Parkinson's disease and heart problems) tend to have low levels of CoQ10. It isn't known which is the chicken and which is the egg or, in other words, whether the disease causes the deficiency or if the deficiency appears first, causing cells to age faster and making disease more likely.

CoQ10 is found in certain foods. The best sources of CoQ10 are oily fish and organ meats, such as beef liver. CoQ10 supplements are available in most pharmacies and health food stores. CoQ10 supplementation may also function as a natural aid in lowering cholesterol and improving heart health, while scant data seem to suggest that it works well in combination with statins. Coenzyme Q10 supplements have few reported side effects. The most common seems to be stomach upset.

CoQ10 can also lower blood sugar levels,[21] although studies

---

[20] https://www.ncbi.nlm.nih.gov/pubmed/15215639
[21] http://www.umm.edu/health/medical/altmed/supplement/coenzyme-q10

on the subject do not seem to be conclusive. Nevertheless, taking CoQ10 supplements may be very important if you are taking statins,[22] because in a consumer update published on February 29, 2012, the FDA warned that statins may increase the risk of type 2 diabetes[23] —something that your doctor may not have bothered to tell you.

CoQ10 supplements can interact with some medications, including beta-blockers, some antidepressants, and chemotherapy drugs. Make sure you consult your doctor before taking CoQ10.

Chromium picolinate – Chromium—specifically, trivalent chromium—is an essential trace element. Chromium forms a compound in the body that seems to enhance the effects of insulin and lower glucose levels. However, it also has risks and its use is somewhat controversial.

A 2014 systematic review and meta-analysis of the efficacy and safety of chromium supplementation in diabetes[24] concluded that "The available evidence suggests favorable effects of chromium supplementation on glycaemic control in patients with diabetes. Chromium monosupplement may additionally improve triglycerides and HDL-C levels. Chromium supplementation at usual doses does not increase the risk of adverse events compared with a placebo. Data on chromium combined supplementation are limited and inconclusive. Long-term benefit and safety of chromium supplementation remain to be further investigated."

A 2015 randomized placebo-controlled trial[25] concluded

---

[22] http://www.lifeextension.com/Magazine/2017/5/Research-Update-Coq10-Fights-Statin-Induced-Diabetes/Page-01

[23] https://www.fda.gov/ForConsumers/ConsumerUpdates/ucm293330.htm

[24] https://www.ncbi.nlm.nih.gov/pubmed/24635480

[25] https://www.ncbi.nlm.nih.gov/pubmed/26406981

that "Four-month treatment with a dietary supplement containing cinnamon, chromium, and carnosine decreased FPG (fasting plasma glucose) and increased fat-free mass in overweight or obese pre-diabetic subjects. These beneficial effects might open up new avenues in the prevention of diabetes."

Another 2015 review of the clinical trial literature[26] concluded that "Cr supplementation with brewer's yeast may provide marginal benefits in lowering FPG in patients with T2DM compared to placebo; however, it did not have any effect on A1C."

Like with other substances (food included), the resulting effect may be very much dependent on your individual response, and that could account for contradictory and inconclusive results in different trials. The conclusion is always the same: you should find out what's good for you, by exploring and testing in a careful and responsible manner. I wouldn't conclude that a supplement is good for you just because it appeared to have a positive effect on somebody else, or even on a large number of people in a medical trial. You could be different in some way that matters to that specific substance.

Probiotics – Probiotics are live bacteria and yeasts that are good for your health, especially your digestive system. Probiotics are often called "good" or "helpful" bacteria because they help keep your gut healthy. Doctors often suggest probiotics to help with digestive problems. Because if you follow the suggestions in this book you will probably be making quite a radical change in your diet, probiotics may help you during the transition period from your original to your new diet.

But are probiotics any good with respect to the management of diabetes? A meta-analysis of randomized trials on the effects

[26] https://www.ncbi.nlm.nih.gov/pubmed/25971249

of probiotics supplement in patients with type 2 diabetes mellitus[27] found that "As a kind of the potential biotherapeutics in the management of T2DM, probiotics can improve glucose control and lipid metabolism." So, at the very least, one can say that probiotics may have a beneficial effect on your digestive system and, perhaps, they can also help manage your blood sugar level.

Fenugreek (Trigonella foenum-graecum) – Fenugreek is a plant that originated from Greece. Studies indicate that fenugreek is useful to normalize the blood sugar level in type 2 diabetes.

One study[28] found that a daily dose of 10 grams of fenugreek seeds soaked in hot water may help control type 2 diabetes. Another study[29] suggests that eating baked goods, such as bread, made with fenugreek flour, may reduce insulin resistance in people with type 2 diabetes.

Fenugreek also has side effects: it can react with several medications, especially with those that treat blood clotting disorders and diabetes. Pregnant women should avoid or limit fenugreek use because of its potential to induce labor. The U.S. Food and Drug Administration (FDA) has not evaluated or approved fenugreek supplements. The manufacturing process is not regulated, so there may be undiscovered health risks. Furthermore, a recent study[30] suggests that fenugreek can cause central hypothyroidism. Therefore, before you decide to use fenugreek you should consult with your doctor also on this point and make sure that you are constantly tested for thyroid activity, to make sure that fenugreek is for you.

[27] https://www.ncbi.nlm.nih.gov/pubmed/28237613
[28] https://www.ncbi.nlm.nih.gov/pubmed/19839001
[29] https://www.ncbi.nlm.nih.gov/pubmed/19857068
[30] https://www.ncbi.nlm.nih.gov/pubmed/28407664

Magnesium – If you exercise strenuously, you may benefit from a magnesium supplement. If you experience leg cramps, particularly at night, you definitely need to consider magnesium supplementation, as that may be a clear sign of magnesium deficiency.

Besides that specific need, magnesium can be beneficial in managing T2D. A 2015 study[31] concluded that oral Mg supplements appear to be useful in persons with T2D to restore Mg deficiencies and to improve insulin resistance, oxidative stress, and systemic inflammation.

Oral Mg supplements have been shown to improve fasting and postprandial glucose levels and insulin sensitivity in hypomagnesemic T2D patients, as well as to improve insulin sensitivity in non-diabetic subjects with insulin resistance.

Many studies have shown that both mean plasma and intracellular free magnesium levels are lower in patients with diabetes than in the general population. This magnesium deficiency, which may take the form of a chronic latent magnesium deficit rather than clinical hypomagnesemia, may have clinical importance because the magnesium ion is a crucial cofactor for many enzymatic reactions involved in metabolic processes. Studies also show that mean plasma levels are lower in patients with both type 1 and type 2 diabetes compared with non-diabetic control subjects.

Unfortunately, testing for magnesium is expensive and not a standard test that your health insurance will happily give you, so you don't know how you are doing with it. Therefore, you should consult with your doctor to see if you can take magnesium supplementation, within the recommended daily intake, to make sure that there is no contraindication for you.

---

[31] https://www.ncbi.nlm.nih.gov/pmc/articles/PMC4549665

Alpha Lipoic Acid – This material is known not so much in regard to glucose level control, but for the purpose of treating neuropathy. In diabetes, "neuropathy" typically refers to nerve damage accumulated over years or decades as a result of increased oxidative stress and reductions in blood flow. When occurring in the extremities (typically the legs and feet), neuropathy can lead to pain, tingling, and numbness. A 2013 study[32] concluded that "Alfa lipoic acid is an effective drug in the treatment of diabetic distal sensory-motor neuropathy and its therapeutic effect is more effective in patients with good glycaemic control."

The reports on alpha lipoic acid are mixed, and there seems to be no real evidence that it helps in reducing glucose level. I am mentioning it here because this material is often brought up in discussions regarding T2D.

Cinnamon – I would avoid using cinnamon to try to reduce blood glucose levels. For one thing, cassia cinnamon, the most common type of cinnamon sold in the United States and Canada, contains varying amounts of coumarin, a substance that may cause or worsen liver disease. And then, while I am not averse to cautiously testing what it makes sense to test, there is little or no conclusive literature pertaining to the effect of cinnamon. A 2013 meta-analysis and systematic review of cinnamon use in type 2 diabetes[33] concluded that "The consumption of cinnamon is associated with a statistically significant decrease in levels of fasting plasma glucose, total cholesterol, LDL-C, and triglyceride levels, and an increase in HDL-C levels; however, no significant effect on hemoglobin A1c was found. The high degree of heterogeneity may limit the ability to apply these results to patient care, because the preferred dose and duration of therapy

---

[32] https://www.ncbi.nlm.nih.gov/pubmed/23678828
[33] https://www.ncbi.nlm.nih.gov/pubmed/24019277

are unclear." This followed a 2012 review,[34] which concluded that "There is insufficient evidence to support the use of cinnamon for type 1 or type 2 diabetes mellitus. Further trials, which address the issues of allocation concealment and blinding, are now required."

---

[34] http://onlinelibrary.wiley.com/doi/10.1002/14651858.CD007170.pub2

CHAPTER 9
Final Words

I am using this chapter to chat with you about some things that didn't fit into the others. These are practical matters that come to my mind when I think of you as someone embarking on this journey without previous experience. Some "good to know" points, nothing more.

Breaking All the Rules

I have said before that you must be strong and adhere strictly to the rules that you will create for yourself. That's right, except that every now and then you need to break the rules and eat bad stuff. You need to do that for two reasons: to remind yourself that you are not missing anything, and to release the pressure that you may feel, because you have been exiled from the dessert table. And then, sometimes you need to celebrate an event and you don't want to watch everybody else drinking that champagne while you make do with tap water. You should aim to do that very seldom, no more than once a month or so, however.

To empower you to break those rules you should talk to your doctor and get a prescription for a glucose-lowering pill that can be taken with food, to avoid hating yourself in the morning when your blood sugar level spikes. Your doctor will likely prescribe metformin for that and you should keep it only for special occasions.

I learned this trick when I was quitting smoking. At first, it was very hard on me, until I decided to buy a pack and keep it in the drawer of my desk. I never opened it, but merely knowing that I had it there and could smoke if I wanted to, made quitting much easier for me. So keep your metformin handy, but don't use it except in emergencies.

Don't Be a Pest

When you start to have sugar-withdrawal symptoms, you are apt to make a pest of yourself with your family. In order to motivate yourself you will apply a good measure of indignation toward the unhealthy foods that your family is eating and will make your diet the central piece of your conversation. Well, don't.

It is true that at that point in time—at least in the first month or so—you need to treat your diet with religious reverence and make sure you are not straying from the right path. But that's you. Your family may not understand what you are doing and may even not believe that you can accomplish what you are trying to do. Besides, it is quite annoying to see you repeatedly refusing a good glass of wine or those juicy potatoes that your spouse had gone to such trouble cooking for you. Understand them. Your transition is hard on them too, because you are changing and we all hate change. The best way to deal with it is to hold your ground politely, without getting into an argument, and to stop talking about it. They'll get used to it when they realize that you mean it.

Maybe You Are Allergic

We recognize that food allergies may have some clear symptoms. Some allergic reactions are annoying but not dangerous, but the most severe allergic reaction is anaphylaxis—a life-threatening whole-body allergic reaction that can impair your breathing, cause a dramatic drop in your blood pressure, and affect your heart rate. Anaphylaxis can come on within minutes of exposure to the trigger food. It can be fatal and must be treated promptly with an injection of epinephrine (adrenaline).

Any food can cause an adverse reaction—write this down: Any Food—but eight types of food account for about 90 percent of all reactions: eggs, milk, peanuts, tree nuts, fish, shellfish, wheat, soy, and certain seeds, including sesame and mustard seeds.

Symptoms of an allergic reaction may involve the skin, the gastrointestinal tract, the cardiovascular system, and the respiratory tract. They can surface in one or more of the following ways: vomiting and/or stomach cramps, hives, shortness of breath, wheezing, repetitive cough, shock or circulatory collapse, tight, hoarse throat, trouble swallowing, swelling of the tongue, affecting the ability to talk or breathe, weak pulse, pale or blue coloring of skin, dizziness or feeling faint, and anaphylaxis.

Yes, and what about high blood sugar level? The fact that this is not a reaction normally considered "allergic" doesn't mean that it is not such. It all depends on how you define "allergic." The *Merriam-Webster Dictionary* defines "allergy" as "a medical condition that causes someone to become sick after eating, touching or breathing something that is harmless to most people." That's you.

The results published by the Weizmann Institute and mentioned in Chapter 2 are an example of why you can have an allergic reaction that results in elevated blood sugar. Some people will have it with white bread and others with whole grain bread. It's individual!

The general wisdom is that eggplant may help reduce blood glucose by inhibiting an enzyme that converts starch to blood sugar. That's cool, except that I know someone who claims that eating eggplant makes his blood sugar go through the roof. I never had a problem eating peanuts, while my daughter gets a migraine at the mere mention of them. That's diversity.

Why am I telling you this? Because you should think of your diet as one that avoids foods that give you an "allergic reaction" resulting in a high blood sugar level. People with celiac disease don't go courting trouble by eating gluten and, similarly, you must avoid foods that trigger an increase in your blood glucose—whether they are generally considered to do so or not. Look at it like that and it may make even more sense to you.

Have We Learned through the Centuries?

What has been will be again,
what has been done will be done again;
there is nothing new under the sun.

[Ecclesiastes 1:9]

When the topic of medical conditions is discussed I often like to consult the 1900 edition of *The Cottage Physician* (see the Appendix) to see how much we have learned in the century and more since then. It is often amazing (and disheartening) to see how little we have advanced and how much we have forgotten. In this case, it is instructive to read the discussion, on page 366, of how to treat diabetes mellitus, and to see how close it is to what I have come up with independently (I only read that page when writing this book). The page is in the appendix, but I am reporting it here for ease of reference:

"Diet must be free from starch and sugar. Exclusive milk diet often benefits. Gluten bread must be substituted for that of wheat flour.[35] Avoid vegetables, arrow-root, asparagus, bread,

---

[35] This seems to be a contradiction but it isn't. Wheat in the year 1900 was nothing like the genetically manipulated brand we have today and was free from its many problems. For a full discussion, refer to Dr. Davis' book.

biscuit, beans, beets, crackers, carrots, macaroni, oat-meal, pastry, potatoes, peas, rice, sago, sugar, tapioca, vermicelli; fruit, apples, grapes, pears, bananas, peaches, plums, pine-apples, raspberries and other sweet fruits; beverages, wine, beer, brandy, also cider and all alcoholic and sweet drinks.

"*Allowable* vegetables, artichokes, cabbage, celery, cresses, cucumbers, olives, greens, lettuce, pickles, mushrooms; fruits, lemons, sour cherries, currants, gooseberries, strawberries and acid fruits, generally; meats, beef, mutton, poultry, game, fish, oysters, cheese, eggs, etc.

"Gratify the thirst by an abundance of good water or skim-milk."

That was 117 years ago. Amazing.

Before We Go

I have done my very best to put all the secrets I have learned in short, useful form, for you to consider and, perhaps, act upon. I sincerely hope that you'll give yourself a chance to get better and, hopefully, to end your dependence on diabetes drugs. There is nothing to be gained by feeding your body with extraneous chemicals if you don't have to, but whether you can be well without them is for you to discover.

My main motivation for writing this book was to give others an opportunity to find their own path out of the vicious circle that T2D and its standard treatment create, and to provide a motivation for doing so. If you find that this book has been of some use to you, please help others to discover it by leaving a review on Amazon or anywhere else where T2D patients may find it.

I do hope that if you accomplish positive results after reading these pages, you'll let me know. I can be reached via my website at www.doitwithwords.com.

Good luck!!

Meet the Author:

Kfir Luzzatto is the author of seven novels, several short stories and three non-fiction books. Kfir was born and raised in Italy, and moved to Israel as a teenager. He acquired the love for the English language from his father, a former U.S. soldier, a voracious reader, and a prolific writer. Kfir has a PhD in chemical engineering and works as a patent attorney. He lives in Omer, Israel, with his full-time partner, Esther, their four children, Michal, Lilach, Tamar, and Yonatan, and the dog Elvis.

Kfir has published extensively in the professional and general press over the years. For almost four years he wrote a weekly "Patents" column in Globes (Israel's financial newspaper). His most recent nonfiction book, *FUN WITH PATENTS—The Irreverent Guide for the Investor, the Entrepreneur and the Inventor*, was published in 2016. He is an HWA (Horror Writers Association) and ITW (International Thriller Writers) member.

Kfir's mind–body web site is www.DoItWithWords.com and you can also visit his literary web site at www.KfirLuzzatto.com.

Follow him on Twitter (@KfirLuzzatto) and on Facebook: https://www.facebook.com/KfirLuzzattoAuthor.

Appendix

The Cottage Physician, 1900

£35
as found
IXSV-DL

THE
Cottage Physician

FOR INDIVIDUAL AND FAMILY USE.

PREVENTION, SYMPTOMS AND TREATMENT.

BEST-KNOWN METHODS

IN ALL

Diseases, Accidents and Emergencies of the Home.

PREPARED BY

The Best Physicians and Surgeons of Modern Practice.

ALLOPATHY, + HOMŒOPATHY,

ETC., ETC.

WITH INTRODUCTION BY

GEORGE W. POST, A.M., M.D.,

Adjunct

Professor of the Practice of Medicine

IN THE

COLLEGE OF PHYSICIANS AND SURGEONS, CHICAGO.

Complete Hand Book of Medical Knowledge for the Home.

NEARLY 200 ILLUSTRATIONS.

The King-Richardson Co.
Springfield, Mass.

RICHMOND. DES MOINES. INDIANAPOLIS. SAN JOSÉ.
DALLAS.   TOLEDO.
1900

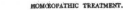

366

Diabetes. (139)—*Uva Ursa*, 1 x, ten drops every three hours in *Diabetes Insipidus*.

Diabetes Mellitus. *Arsenicum*, 3 x, very hungry and thirsty; pale skin; loss of strength; dryness of mouth and throat; excessive urination; watery diarrhœa.

Phosphoric Acid, 1 x, loss of nerve force, with frequent urination. Diet must be free from starch and sugar. Exclusive milk diet often benefits. Gluten bread must be substituted for that of wheat flour. Avoid vegetables, arrow-root, asparagus, bread, biscuit, beans, beets, crackers, carrots, macaroni, oat-meal, pastry, potatoes, peas, rice, sago, sugar, tapioca, vermicelli; fruit, apples, grapes, pears, bananas, peaches, plums, pine-apples, raspberries and other sweet fruits; beverages, wine, beer, brandy, also cider and all alcoholic and sweet drinks.

Allowable vegetables, artichokes, cabbage, celery, cresses, cucumbers, olives, greens, lettuce, pickles, mushrooms; fruits, lemons, sour cherries, currants, gooseberries, strawberries and acid fruits, generally; meats, beef, mutton, poultry, game, fish, oysters, cheese, eggs, etc.

Gratify the thirst by an abundance of good water or skim-milk. The diabetic should be warmly clad.

Diarrhœa. (140)—*Camphor* φ, sudden diarrhœa with chilliness.

Dulcamara, 3 x, diarrhœa caused from getting wet; worse at night, bilious stools.

China, 1 x, painless, summer diarrhœa.

Chamomilla, 30, diarrhœa in children, accompanying teething.

Arsenicum, 3 x, chronic diarrhœa; red, burning tongue; vomits—even a small amount of water, in fact, everything taken into the stomach.

Ipecac, 1 x, diarrhœa and dysentery accompanied by much nausea.

Veratrum Alb., 1 x, vomiting and diarrhœa attended with cold sweating; cholera morbus; cholera infantum.

Avoid all animal food during an attack of diarrhœa. A little brandy may be added to milk with benefit.

Dilation of the Heart. (142)—*Digitaline*, 3 x, will strengthen a weak heart.

Phosphorus, 3 x, valuable as a tonic, giving tone to the system.

Diphtheria. (143)—Call your physician. *Apis Mel.*, 3 x, in diphtheria with much swelling of the throat, internally, and a stinging pain.

78022021R00043

Made in the USA
Middletown, DE
28 June 2018